Contents

KU-319-987

Preface

The aim of treatment of diabetes is not only to restore the patient to health, but also to enable him or her to aspire to a normal lifespan free from diabetes-related disablement.

This book, intended primarily for medical students, junior hospital staff and general practitioners, has been written to help those concerned in the care of diabetics to understand the home, laboratory and ward side-room tests that are the essential accompaniment to successful control of the disease.

Laboratory and side-room tests vary in their level of complexity: we have therefore attempted to give an assessment of the amount of information that can be obtained with equipment of different degrees of sophistication, ranging from visual assessment of colour change to microprocessor-controlled equipment, in order to cover facilities likely to be available in services of widely differing affluence. Some of the tests described are simple manual procedures requiring the minimum of expensive equipment. They are included in this book to show how useful analytical results can be obtained with limited resources, either in the absence of sophisticated laboratory facilities, or where such facilities are too distant from the ill patient to be of immediate use.

1   **2**

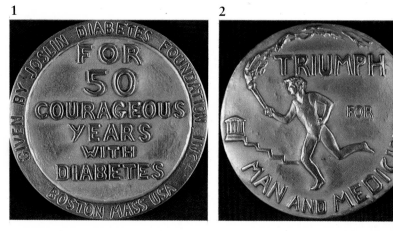

1 and 2 Joslin Diabetes Foundation Bronze Medal. This particular medal was awarded to Mrs Mary Fraser of Aberdeen in October 1977 for 50 years of healthy life as an insulin-dependent diabetic.

Clinical Tests

Diabetes Mellitus
Laboratory tests and self-monitoring

B. J. Boucher, MD, FRCP
Consultant Physician, The London Hospital
Senior Lecturer, Medical Unit,
The London Hospital Medical College

Iain S. Ross, MB, Ph.D
Consultant in Charge, Clinical Biochemistry,
Grampian Health Board
Senior Lecturer, University of Aberdeen

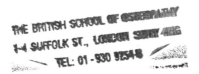
Wolfe Medical Publications Ltd

General Editor, Wolfe Tests Series
D. Geraint James MA, MD (Cantab.), FRCP (London)

This book is one of the titles in the series of Wolfe Medical Atlases, a series which brings together probably the world's largest systematic published collection of diagnostic colour photographs.
    For a full list of atlases in the series, plus forthcoming titles and details of our surgical, dental and veterinary atlases, please write to Wolfe Medical Publications Ltd, 2–16 Torrington Place, London WC1E 7LT.

1. Introduction

Diabetes mellitus is a condition in which blood glucose levels rise as a result of inadequate insulin action. It appears to have many causes. Complications of this syndrome include damage to tissues such as the retina and lens in the eye, the kidneys and nerves. Worsening of atheromatous disease in large blood vessels may also occur. Despite the introduction of insulin more than 50 years ago, these complications have remained very common in diabetes, causing serious disabilities and early death. The risk of complications increases with the duration of the disease.

Since the late 1970s it has become apparent that the rate of progression of some complications can be ameliorated by meticulous long-term control of diabetes as judged simply by control of glycaemia. Tests are required so that day-to-day adjustment of treatment can be made in order to achieve near-normoglycaemia without danger of hypoglycaemia, and are also useful in the long term to detect those 'well' diabetics with poor glycaemic control as soon as possible. Assessment of the ill diabetic remains necessary so that ketoacidosis and similar metabolic crises can be spotted early, diagnosed correctly and managed safely.

Almost all the laboratory tests used in the assessment of diabetes depend on blood samples, though urine can be used in some. Blood sampling is obviously unpleasant, and increases the number of needle punctures for those diabetics who already have to inject insulin. It is important, therefore, that the problems of blood sampling are kept to a minimum for patients whose condition will last for life. Venous blood should be drawn only when no smaller sample will do, and then it should be done by experts.

Capillary blood is increasingly used both in hospital and by patients for self-monitoring at home. Care must be taken to use, and to teach patients to use, safe, clean and comfortable 'stick' techniques. The lower ear lobe rim can be used as a puncture site as it is less sensitive and less likely to become dirty afterwards than is the tip of the finger. A mirror is the only extra gadget one needs to prick one's own ear lobe. Fingerpricks, however, are widely used. They are less likely to be painful or to become infected if done on the outer edge of the pulp. Holding the thumb and chosen fingertip lightly together leaves a rim of exposed fingertip laterally that can easily be used for puncture. Spirit may be used to clean the skin but must be allowed to dry before inserting the needle, a) because it stings, and b) because it spoils capillary test results. Cleansing with spirit is normally necessary only when testing in 'dirty' places, such as hospitals!

Those taking blood or teaching self-monitoring must regard all blood drawn as potentially hazardous in view of the many diseases fresh blood can transmit (including hepatitis B and AIDS) and all material used in testing, including test sticks, must be disposed of in suitable containers for burning.

2. Urine testing

Glycosuria

Urine testing is widely used to screen for diabetes mellitus as it is easy, cheap and noninvasive. The absence of sugar(s) from the urine does not, however, exclude diabetes, as the urinary glucose threshold is above the normal blood glucose level and rises with age. Similarly, sugar in the urine does not necessarily mean that diabetes mellitus is present. Beginning treatment (other than dietary avoidance of simple sugars) without confirmation of the diagnosis by blood tests can therefore be dangerous.

Urine testing is the usual method of monitoring diabetic control as it does give some idea of blood glucose levels. However, home monitoring of blood glucose levels is increasingly being used in an attempt to achieve near-normoglycaemia. Urine testing is also used in well-controlled diabetics with a normal renal threshold for glucose as a marker of loss of control.

Chemical tests for detection of glycosuria

All familiar tests for the chemical detection of glycosuria depend upon the reduction of copper salts. The blue-coloured copper ion reacts with the reducing substance in the urine and forms red copper oxide. The interaction of colours between the blue non-reduced copper salt and the red copper oxide gives a range of colours from blue to green to yellow to orange to brown. Tests based on liquid reagents such as Fehling's and Benedict's have now universally been replaced by reagents in tablet form (3). The tablets consist of copper sulphate, sodium carbonate, sodium hydroxide and citric acid.

$$\underset{\text{(Blue)}\;\text{NaOH}}{\overset{\text{Cu\;citrate}}{\longrightarrow}}\;\text{Cu -citrate complex}$$

$$\underset{\text{NaOH}}{\overset{\text{Glucose}}{\longrightarrow}}\;\text{CuOH}\longrightarrow\;\underset{\text{(Red)}}{Cu_2O}\downarrow$$

The tablets are supplied with a test tube and standard dropper. Five drops of urine are placed in the test tube and, using the same dropper, 10

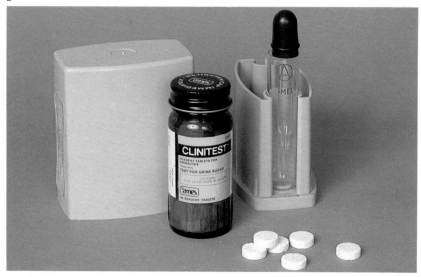

3   Copper reduction test in tablet form for urinary reducing substances.

drops of water are added. A tablet is added to the mixture. Intense heat and effervescence are produced. Fifteen seconds after the effervescence is ended the mixture is shaken and the colour compared with the manu-facturer's colour chart. If an orange colour appears during the effer-vescence but immediately changes to brown, more than 2 g% of glucose is present. It is therefore essential to observe the colour change throughout the reaction process.

Sensitivity
The lower level of sensitivity has been reported to be 150 mg of glucose per 100 ml. Using the standard technique, the upper level of semi-quantitative determination is 2 g%, but this can be increased by repeating the test on a modified dilution schedule.

Specificity
This test is based on the reducing properties of glucose. Other reducing substances can be present in urine, for example:

Reducing carbohydrates	Non-carbohydrate reducing substances
Lactose	Ascorbic acid
Fructose	Chloral hydrate
Galactose	Glucuronic acid
Pentoses	Conjugates of isoniazid
	Tetracycline
	Streptomycin
	Penicillin
	Salicylates
	Acetylsalicylates
	Formaldehyde

All the above substances give the characteristic colour reaction described for glucose. Occasionally, blackish colours are produced by a reaction with excreted radio-opaque contrast medium or some antibiotics. The black colour is unmistakable but could mask the more normal colours produced by glucose.

The tablet test is relatively reliable in giving an assessment to the nearest ½% of reducing substances present in urine, but it requires a source of clean water, a safe place for the disposal of the highly caustic products of the reaction, and a safe, dry place for the storage of the tablets. The tablets, if swallowed, can cause severe oesophageal and gastric ulceration. These limitations probably mean that this form of test is now approaching the end of its useful life.

Detection of glycosuria via enzyme strip
The most useful method of detecting glucose in urine is to use enzymatic test paper. Glucose oxidase is a plant enzyme that oxidises glucose selectively to gluconic acid. Hydrogen peroxide is formed. In all rapid enzymatic tests the hydrogen peroxide so formed is detected by means of a colour reaction, usually produced by the activity of a peroxidase.

$$\beta\text{-D-glucose} + O_2 \xrightarrow{\text{glucose oxidase}} \text{gluconic acid} + H_2O_2$$

$$H_2O_2 + \underset{\text{(Colourless)}}{\text{chromogen}} \xrightarrow{\text{peroxidase}} H_2O + \underset{\text{(Coloured)}}{\text{oxidised chromogen}}$$

Several commercial versions of the enzymatic dipstick test are available, the reaction being similar in all. The reactive end of the strip is dipped briefly in collected urine, or held briefly in the stream of urine. Surplus urine is carefully wiped or shaken off. After a measured time ($\frac{1}{2}$ to 2 minutes depending upon the make of stick) the test area is compared with a scale of colours on the packet (**4** and **5**).

Sensitivity
Theoretically, sensitivity is very high, with detection in a distilled water system as low as 5 mg% glucose, however as urine contains a number of physiological inhibitors, an approximate lower level of sensitivity of 80 mg% is the most commonly quoted value (similar to that of Benedict's chemical test).

Specificity
As the first step in the reaction involves the enzyme glucose oxidase, it has virtually absolute specificity for glucose. Nonspecific positive results are, however, possible with the colour complexing step as this is not specific. In addition, as the reaction is enzyme mediated, extremes of pH can overcome the buffering system and inhibit or enhance the enzyme. The system is also temperature dependent, the reaction being slowed when urine specimens have been refrigerated (see chapter on blood monitoring).

The final colour reaction on many of the enzyme strips is sufficiently well graded to enable a semi-quantitative assessment to be made of the amount of glucose present in the urine.

The strips are stable if kept dry and do not require careful measuring or disposal, nor are they themselves chemically dangerous. They are therefore to be preferred in the semi-quantitative estimation of glucose in the urine. Note also that at the time of writing, urine dipsticks are one-tenth the price of blood dipsticks.

4 Enzyme-based urine strip test for glucose. This particular brand uses two pads per strip to give wide sensitivity. Note the colour change between the fresh and the reacted strip.

5 Single-pad type enzyme-based urine dip test showing the used strip being compared with the colour chart printed on the container.

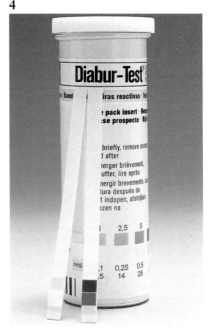

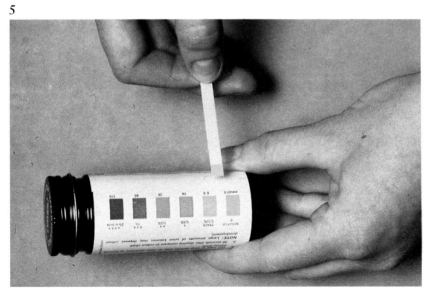

Ketonuria

Examination of the urine for ketones provides a simple and sensitive test for the presence of ketosis (if deficiency of carbohydrate intake can be excluded) in the diabetic, and is widely used. These tests should be used by patients who are liable to acute upsets in control and by doctors who may need to decide whether a diabetic is becoming ill.

Three ketone bodies are present in the urine. Acetoacetate is the parent compound, the reduction of which gives ß-hydroxybutyrate and its decarboxylation yields acetone.

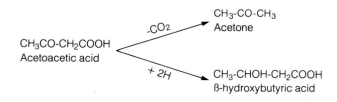

These three substances always occur together in the urine (the ratio of acetone to acetoacetic acid is about 1:10): it is therefore sufficient to detect acetoacetic acid, which occurs in the greatest amount. There is no clear correlation between ketonuria and the ketone content of blood: this means that very high levels of ketonuria can be detected in the case of starvation ketosis with only slight ketonaemia being present. In keto-acidotic coma, however, ketone excretion is inevitable, provided renal function is preserved.

Both strip and tablet tests are available for the detection of ketonuria. Both are developments of the same basic nitroprusside reaction. The exact mechanism of the reaction is uncertain, but one suggestion is described below. (R = CH_3 for acetone or = CH_2COOH for acetoacetic acid.)

$$Na_2[fe(CN)_5 NO] + CH_3CO\text{-}R + NAOH$$
(Colourless)

$$\downarrow$$

$$Na_3[fe(CN)_5 \, N = CH\text{-}CO\text{-}R] + H_2O$$
$$\underset{\text{(Violet blue)}}{\overset{|}{OH}}$$

ß-ketones and other substances with an enolysable keto group react in this way, but ß-hydroxybutyrate does not react.

Ketone-sensitive tablets

The tablets contain sodium nitroprusside, glycine, disodium phosphate and lactose. (The lactose is present to accentuate the staining.)

One tablet is moistened with a drop of urine; after 30 seconds a comparison is made of the violet colour seen on the tablet with the colour scale provided by the manufacturers.

Sensitivity

Comparison colour	Acetoacetic acid mg/100 ml	Acetone mg/100 ml
Weak	10 to 20	25 to 50
Average	25 to 40	200 to 250
Strong	over 50	400 to 1000

Specificity

The nitroprusside reaction is not highly specific, but acetoacetic acid and acetone are virtually the only substances with an enolysable keto group that occur in urine. One exception is phenylpyruvic acid, which occurs in untreated cases of phenylketonuria. Large concentrations of phenyl-pyruvic acid give an orange/brown colour, which will not be confused with the violet colour of a positive acetone reaction.

A faint positive is sometimes possible with the urine of patients being treated with large doses of L-dopa.

It is sometimes possible to obtain a sudden colour change on the tablet when colourless potential pigments passed in the urine suddenly develop colour on contact with the alkaline buffer in the tablet (e.g. bromsulfophthalein). That this is a false positive reaction is detectable because the colour change is instant and not gradual as is the reaction with acetoacetate and acetone.

Stability

The tablets are very sensitive to dampness and should be kept in a tightly stoppered bottle, preferably with desiccant.

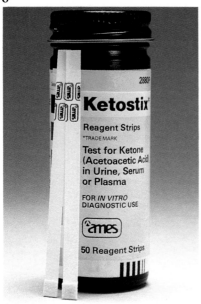

6 Ketone-sensitive urine strip test showing fresh and reacted colour pads.

Ketone-sensitive stick tests (6)
These test strips are also based on the nitroprusside reaction. The sticks are dipped in the urine and after a timed delay the colour change is read against the chart provided by the manufacturer.

Sensitivity
Sensitivity is slightly different to that obtained with the tablet test and is therefore shown here:

Comparison colour	Acetoacetic acid mg/100 ml	Acetone mg/100 ml
Weak	10 to 20	80 to 140
Moderate	30 to 50	320 to 820
Strong	80 to 120	1600 to 2400

Specificity
Interfering substances are similar to those noted for the tablet test, and the sticks are also very sensitive to dampness and should be kept dry in a well-stoppered bottle.

Proteinuria

The presence of protein in the urine of diabetics as detected by simple bedside tests may indicate urinary tract infection or a vaginal discharge, but when it persists in the absence of pus cells it usually reflects the onset of irreversible renal damage. Now that renal replacement is increasingly feasible in the diabetic this is a useful screening test for checking on renal function.

The detection of protein in urine is often arbitrarily divided into two levels of sensitivity: proteinuria (or albuminuria) and microproteinuria (or microalbuminuria).

Detection of proteinuria (albuminuria)
There is no tablet for the detection of proteinuria and all the test papers depend upon the principle of the protein error of an indicator. This was first described using the potassium salt of tetrabromophenolphthalein. In acid, this indicator is present in a yellow form. Proteins can form salt-like blue compounds from which they are not displaced by hydrogen ions. If the acid pH remains the same, proteins can thus cause a 'false' change in the indicator colour, which is observed as a protein error. This phenomenon is seen with many indicators, but particularly with compounds of the tetrabromophthalein series.

Individual test paper manufacturers differ in their use of indicators, and in some cases use mixed indicators.

The test strip is dipped into the urine, removed quickly, and wiped on the side of the vessel. After 10 seconds the colour change (if any) is compared with the colour scale provided by the manufacturer. The scale goes from negative to 10 g/l in four steps.

Sensitivity
In most of the stick tests the lower level of sensitivity is 150 to 200 mg/l, as albumin.

The protein error method is markedly dependent on the number of free amino groups of the individual protein fractions; therefore with different proteins the degree of colour change will vary. By far the strongest colour change is seen with albumin. There is a much weaker reaction for globulins, glycoproteins and mucoproteins. Bence Jones proteins show practically no protein error.

Specificity
The test is not specific for any particular group of proteins or proteins in general, however it rarely misleads if fresh urine is used. If the urine is

contaminated with acid, or if it is stale to the extent that contaminant bacteria have markedly changed the pH of the urine, then the buffer in the test strip can be overcome and the indicator will react to the pH of the urine. However, if fresh urine is used and the manufacturer's instructions are followed carefully, it is reasonably protein-specific.

Multiple test strips

Urine sticks with glucose-, ketone- and albumin-sensitive pads on the same strip are useful in diabetic clinics and hospital wards (7). They are less costly than carrying out three individual strip tests on the urine, but if the tester does not require the three pieces of information then obviously they are more expensive than carrying out specific single tests. It is not usually necessary, therefore, to use these sticks outside the specialist clinic or hospital ward. However, a stick that combines glucose- and ketone-sensitive pads can be used at home where both tests are required in unstable diabetics (8).

Detection of microproteinuria (microalbuminuria)

These terms are used to describe proteinuria present below the level of concentration detectable by dipstick methods, that is, below 200 mg/l. Microproteinuria is a very sensitive indicator of early renal damage, and it is likely that it relates to reversible damage. Therefore it is necessary to consider testing for microproteinuria as part of the routine monitoring of diabetics, as its presence is as useful a marker of high risk of serious complications. Thus it may be possible to prevent deterioration in some patients.

Most urine contains trace amounts of protein, the reference range for normals being quoted as up to 10 or 12 mg/l. Methods of testing for microproteinuria would therefore need to have a range of detection between 10 mg/l and 200 mg/l. This is possible only with laboratory-based tests at present, for example radioimmunoassay or nepheloimmunoassay. The results can be expressed either as the amount of protein per litre or the amount of protein passed over a timed period of urine collection.

Laboratory tests for microproteinuria

Several laboratory methods are available with the sensitivity to detect protein levels from 10 to 100 mg/l. Most of the well-established methods are radioimmunoassays for albumin. However, it would greatly assist in the assessment of diabetics if a method was readily available at low cost that did not involve the use of radioactive tracers. Modern high-sensitivity

7 Urine dipstick with pads sensitive to protein, glucose and ketones. This is useful for screening of urine in a diabetic clinic or hospital ward.

8 Urine dipstick with pads sensitive to glucose and ketones. These strips are of use for unstable, ketosis-prone diabetics to use at home.

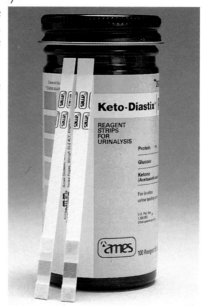

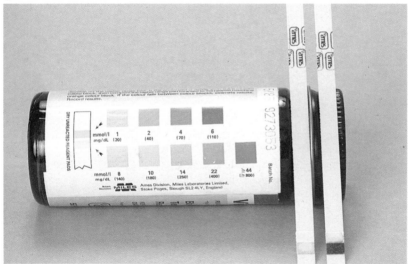

nephelometric techniques for detection of albumin at this level are being developed.

Once the presence of low levels of albumin is detected in the urine it becomes important to follow the results of therapeutic intervention. This means that it is necessary not only to detect the presence of albumin but also to quantify any change in its excretion rate. The albumin level therefore has to relate either to the excretion rate (i.e. milligrams per 24 hours) or to a stable constituent in urine, such as creatinine. The collection of a timed urine sample is difficult and in the first instance it is recommended that albumin excretion is expressed as a protein/creatinine ratio in an early morning or a daytime specimen from the patient (albumin excretion rates vary as to whether the patient is recumbent or ambulent). The use of a random access analyser for these procedures renders it easy to analyse a urine specimen for microalbumin and creatinine within the service of a general clinical chemistry laboratory, without the special precautions necessary when handling radioactive tracers.

Urinary tract infections

Sepsis, both acute and chronic, is quite common in diabetics. Proteinuria may be the first indication of such sepsis and its detection should be followed by immediate examination of fresh urine for pus cells and bacteria, as well as for casts, which would reflect nephritic damage without sepsis.

Dipstick tests for bacteria, based on the detection of urinary nitrite, are available. Urine culture, with identification of any organism and its antibiotic sensitivity, is useful in guiding treatment in acute sepsis and essential if tuberculosis is suspected, as organisms cannot always be seen in the urine. Six-week cultures are needed for its detection if more rapid chemical detection using high performance liquid chromatography (HPLC) is not available.

The detection of urinary tract infection by urine culture and testing for antibiotic sensitivity remains a laboratory-based procedure. This is the definitive method of confirming and characterising urinary tract infections, however there are two non-laboratory-based methods which can assist in detecting asymptomatic urinary tract infection in patients: measurement of urinary nitrate and excess leukocytes.

Detection of urinary nitrite
Urine provides a natural culture medium for a great variety of organisms, however, most cases of urinary tract infection are caused by *Escherichia coli* derived from the patient's own gastrointestinal tract.

About 100 years ago Grice introduced a test to detect nitrite in urine. Nitrite is produced by many strains of bacteria which, when present in excess in urine, break down the nitrate normally present. The nitrite is detected by forming a diazonium compound in an acid solution with the nitrite. This is then coupled to give a coloured product. For example, in one nitrite test, an aromatic amine sulphanilamide is reacted to form a red azo dye. The reaction is easily presented in an impregnated paper strip form.

Sensitivity
When interpreting the test it is necessary to have allowed the urine to remain in the bladder long enough to give any bacteria present time to act upon the nitrate. It is therefore essential that the test is carried out after at least 4 to 6 hours of bladder incubation. This is most conveniently done by instructing the patient to collect the first early morning specimen of urine, which has been in the bladder overnight. When such precautions are taken it has been claimed that the test can detect over 70% of significant bacteriurias.

Occasionally, the bacteria in the urine are not nitrate-splitting organisms. This will obviously give a false negative result, but this is not a common phenomenon.

Specificity
The test is specific for nitrite, which is normally present in large amounts in the urine only as a consequence of significant bacterial action. Not enough nitrite is excreted from normal food sources to cause the test to be positive.

Detection of excess leukocytes in urine
A recent introduction is a dipstick urine test for the detection of leukocyte esterase. The products of enzyme action on leukocyte esterase are linked with an indicator system which will cause a colour change on an impregnated strip. It is claimed that the test is not affected by the bacteria present in the urine, nor by erythrocyte concentrations of up to 100,000 per µl. The colour that develops after 60 seconds on the impregnated paper strip is said to be equivalent to 10 to 25 leukocytes per µl. As yet, it is not known to what extent this test is more sensitive in detecting urinary tract infection than the cheaper nitrite test.

The use of both of the above-mentioned strip tests makes it possible to detect a significant number of urinary tract infections without the difficulties of urinary preservation and the cost of detailed laboratory analysis.

However, once infection has been indicated by these methods it is necessary to send a specimen to the laboratory for culture and sensitivity to antibiotics.

3. Blood sugars

Glucose is metabolically the most important sugar in the blood: it is an essential fuel and is involved in energy provision and metabolism. Estimation of sugar levels by methods that assess total reducing sugars will measure both glucose and other sugars (fructose, ribose, etc.). Normally, non-glucose sugars are present in smaller amounts. In some congenital metabolic defects interference by non-glucose sugars can prevent recognition of hypoglycaemia, and specific enzyme methods are therefore valuable in the diagnosis of hypoglycaemia, especially in young children.

Good diabetic care requires reasonably precise blood sugar/glucose measurements. Precise laboratory estimates of blood glucose are useful for diagnostic blood tests and glucose tolerance testing (Table 1), however, a simple test with immediate results is of great value in the known diabetic (whether on insulin or not) so that hypoglycaemic therapy can be adjusted appropriately. For this reason, methods that can be used by doctor, nurse and patients themselves are widely used, even though their precision can be somewhat less than that of standard laboratory estimations.

Table 1 The World Health Organisation guidelines on interpretation of oral glucose tolerance test (1985).
Glucose load for adults: 75 g in 250 to 350 ml of water.
Glucose load for children: 1.75 g per kg of body weight to a maximum dose of 75 g.

| | Glucose concentration, mmol/l | | | |
| | Whole blood | | Plasma | |
	Venous	Capillary	Venous	Capillary
Diabetes mellitus				
Fasting value	≥ 6.7	≥ 6.7	≥ 7.8	≥ 7.8
2 h after glucose load	≥10.0	≥11.1	≥11.1	≥12.2
Impaired glucose tolerance				
Fasting value	< 6.7	< 6.7	< 7.8	< 7.8
2 h after glucose load	6.7 to 10.0	7.8 to 11.1	7.8 to 11.1	8.9 to 12.2

Analytical methods

Factors affecting the results

a) Physiological factors

i) *Blood vs plasma.* The concentration of glucose present in the plasma water and cell water is the same, but because of the lower water content of the cells (73% vs 93%) plasma glucose is higher than total blood glucose. This difference amounts to approximately 12% if the patient has a normal haematocrit, and for each change in the haematocrit of 10 units there is a change in the opposite direction of blood glucose of 0.20 mmol/l (3.6 mg%).

ii) *Arterial vs venous sample.* There is little difference in glucose concentration between arterial (capillary) and venous blood if the patient is fasting, however at the post-prandial peak glucose is higher on the arterial side by up to 1.9 mmol/l (35 mg%). This differential is caused by the use of carbohydrate as a fuel in post-prandial metabolism.

b) Methodological factors

Reducing vs enzymatic. When glucose is measured by its reducing property the value obtained also includes other reducing substances (see page 9). These substances contribute to a greater extent to the analytical result when whole blood is used, as there is then an additional contribution from red cell glutathione. Other reducing substances are present in small amounts in both cells and plasma.

Reducing methods

Historically, the best known reaction for reducing substances in blood is that of Nelson–Somogyi.

$$\text{Glucose} + Cu^{2+} + OH^- \xrightarrow[100°C]{} \text{mixed sugar acids} + Cu_2O \text{ (complexed to give coloured product)}$$

Nelson–Somogyi methodology has now been supplanted by a method using ortho-toluidine as this does not react with non-glucose reducing substances in blood. Ortho-toluidine reacts quantitatively with the aldehyde group of aldohexoses. Thus, in the absence of large amounts of lactose, etc., it is reasonably specific for glucose.

PRINCIPLE

Ortho-toluidine + glucose

Read at 620 to 630 nm
(Schiff base)

Manual	Automated
Sample: 200 µl whole blood or 50 µl plasma. *Equipment:* Centrifuge, boiling water, bath, colorimeter at 620 nm. *Comment:* Accuracy fair. Precision is dependent on analyst. *References:* Cooper and McDaniel 1970; Dubowski 1962.	*Sample:* 200 µl whole blood. *Equipment:* Continuous flow modules – sample, pump, 100°C oil bath, colorimeter at 620 nm, recorder. *Comment:* Accuracy fair. Precision good. *Reference:* Winkers and Jacob 1971.

Manual or automated methods can be used with capillary samples.

Glucose oxidase methods

In these methods the aldehyde group of glucose is oxidised by glucose oxidase to give gluconic acid, with gluconolactone as intermediate. The glucose oxidase (GOD) reaction is specific but can be inhibited by fluoride in excess. The oxygen consumption in the GOD reaction or subsequent peroxidase colour complexing is not specific and is subject to positive and negative interference. Used carefully, however, glucose oxidase methods can give results very close to true glucose levels, and are particularly recommended for detecting hypoglycaemic states. In all circumstances plasma is the preferred sample. As this is an enzyme reaction it is temperature-dependent and therefore requires good temperature stability.

PRINCIPLE

$$\text{Glucose} + H_2O + O_2 \xrightarrow[\text{oxidase}]{\text{glucose}} \text{gluconic acid } H_2O_2$$

$$\text{Colourless } O_2 \text{ acceptor} + H_2O_2 \xrightarrow{\text{peroxidase}} H_2O + O_2 + \text{coloured oxidised acceptor}$$

Oxygen acceptor system of Trinder = phenol + 4-aminophenazone

Manual

Sample:
100 µl whole blood.

Equipment:
Centrifuge, 37°C bath, colorimeter at 515 nm.

Comment:
Accuracy good. Precision is dependent on analyst.

Reference:
Trinder 1969.

Automated

Macro sample:
100 µl whole blood.

Semimicro:
50 µl whole blood.

Equipment:
Continuous flow modules: sampler, pump, dialyser, 37°C heating bath, colorimeter at 505 nm, recorder.

Comment:
Accuracy good. Precision good.

Reference:
Richardson 1977.

Discrete micro methods

Sample:
5 µl plasma, up to 25 µl whole blood.

Oxygen consumed in the glucose oxidase reaction is measured polarographically.

Comment:
Accuracy good. Precision good with careful analyst.

Reference:
Kadish, Little and Sternberg 1968.

Non-laboratory methods of blood glucose collection and estimation

Capillary blood collected by the patient from a finger or ear lobe, or collected by the nurse or clinic attendant from the same sites, can be sent to the laboratory, suitably stabilised for later analysis, or, using one of the dried reagent strip test systems (BG strips), analysed at the time of collection.

Using BG strips, the patient or attendant can either quantify the result visually by comparing the colour change on the strip against the manufacturer's colour chart (similar to urine testing); or the strip can be sent to the nearest clinic or laboratory for assessment; or it can be read in one of the small battery-powered reflectance meters (see 27 to 30).

The unit cost of the technically sophisticated reagent strip systems is often higher than that of a laboratory wet chemistry system, and some of the special packages designed to transport a capillary blood sample to the laboratory for analysis can also be relatively expensive. Therefore the use of a non-laboratory-based method of blood collection and analysis should be carefully assessed, and used only where the laboratory facility is not available or would produce unacceptable delay, or when the clinical value of an immediate result is clear.

Methods of collecting a capillary blood sample and the means by which the samples can be analysed are shown on the following pages.

How to obtain a capillary blood sample

9

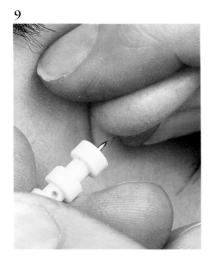

9 It is recommended that the ear lobe is used as a puncture site as it is usually easily manipulated, it is cleaner than the hand, it has thinner keratin, and it is much less sensitive. In children there is the added advantage that the ear stab and the blood drop cannot be seen. Finger or earlobe should be warm and squeezed gently to obtain a large drop of blood.

10

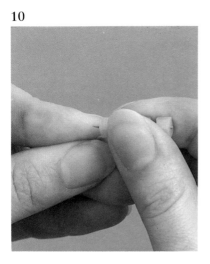

10 Sample obtained from the finger by the patient. Hands should be washed and carefully dried. If the skin around the stab wound is wet, blood may lyse and give misleading results. The side of the finger usually has thinner keratin than the central area. A spring-loaded stilette holder (**11** and **12**) can help the nervous or uncertain patient to learn the technique but this is not a necessity. A clean disposable lancet is essential. It should be used once only.

DO NOT ATTEMPT TO USE A SMALL DROP OF BLOOD. IT WILL GIVE MISLEADING RESULTS.

11 A selection of spring-loaded stilettes. These can help a nervous patient obtain a good capillary blood sample.

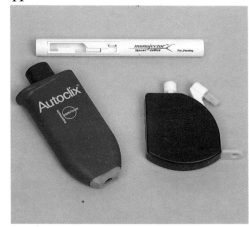

12 Spring-loaded stilette used for a finger stab.

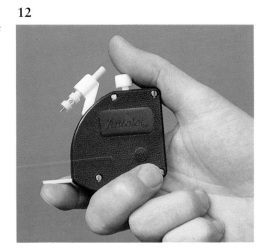

Collecting the sample

No attempt should be made to collect the sample until a drop of blood of sufficient size has been produced on the finger or ear lobe (**13** and **14**). Whether the sample is being collected for future analysis or applied to one of the reagent test strips, it should be collected with the minimum amount of smearing and without contact with either water or other potential lysing agents such as swab alcohol.

13   **14**

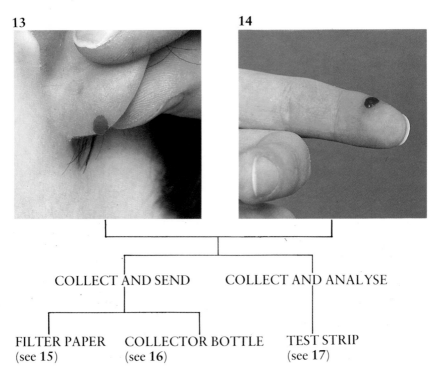

COLLECT AND SEND   COLLECT AND ANALYSE

FILTER PAPER   COLLECTOR BOTTLE   TEST STRIP
(see **15**)   (see **16**)   (see **17**)

15 Filter paper. The drop of blood should be applied to the centre of each circle, so that the circle is seen to be filled through the full depth of the paper. The spot, labelled with the date and time of collection, is allowed to dry at room temperature. The card can represent a series of timed and dated specimens as advised by the doctor (Gamelon 1982).

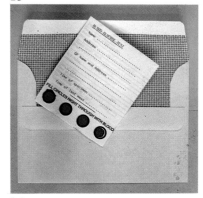

16 Collector bottles. The top of the collector bottle should be removed and the ring round the neck of the bottle discarded. Blood should be gently scraped into the small cup-like depression in the top of the collector. This cup should be filled (5 μl). The top of the collection bottle is then firmly screwed back on and the entire bottle given a sharp tap. The small collector well will then drop into the preservative and the sample will be stable for posting to the laboratory for analysis. The analysis involves adaptation of standard laboratory methods.

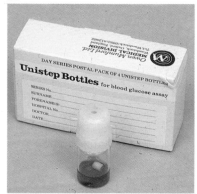

17 Test strip. At the time of application a watch with a second hand, a digital watch, or an accurate timer should be available. The blood drop should cover most of the test pad or pads with a generous layer. The strip can be moved around to spread the blood over the pads. Smearing of blood thinly over the strips will not provide sufficient liquid to give a valid result. The blood should be allowed to remain in contact with the strip for the exact time specified by the manufacturer.

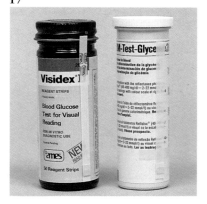

Use of reagent strip tests (BG strips) – essential points

1 BG strips are a highly sophisticated chemical system based on enzymes. They should therefore be stored with desiccant. It is advisable to keep the strips in a refrigerator for long-term storage, but on no account should the strips be used straight from the fridge. Any enzyme system is usually temperature-dependent and erroneous results will be obtained from strips used before they have equilibrated to the ambient temperature.

2 The size of the blood drop must be sufficiently large to wet the reagent thoroughly and to cover a sufficient area to enable the colour change to be easily seen (**18** to **22**).

18   **19**

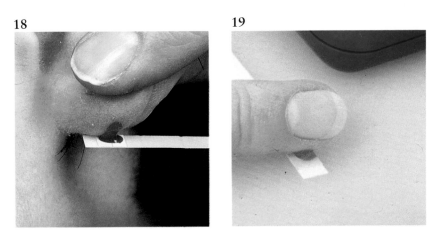

18 and 19   **Ear and finger capillary blood samples are applied to the BG strip.** The size of the drop must be sufficiently large.

20

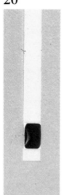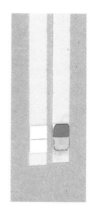

20   A good-sized drop of blood results in a good, even colour reaction across a large area of the strip, which is easily read visually or in a reflectance meter.

21

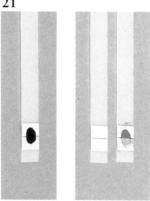

21   A drop of blood that is too small will give an insufficient reaction area on the strip, making it difficult to read visually. It also increases the edge effect of dried blood round the small reacted area.

22

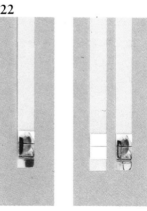

22   A smeared sample often dries on the pad and cannot be wiped off – a useless test.

3   The duration of contact of the blood drop with the strip must be very carefully and accurately timed (**23**). Colour development is not linear and therefore a halving or a doubling of the blood contact or colour development time does not increase the sensitivity nor extend the range of the strip.

4   The removal of the blood drop from the reagent pad is accomplished either by careful wiping (or by washing off with a stream of water) as advised by the manufacturers (**24** and **25**). BG strips that need wiping are much preferred as this reduces the likelihood of contamination.

5   Following use, if the stick is dry, the colours remain reasonably stable and therefore can be sent by post to the nearest hospital or laboratory for checking, or can be kept to be seen by a visiting nurse or doctor (**26**). If the sticks are to be kept it is essential that they are placed in a receptacle with a desiccant.

23

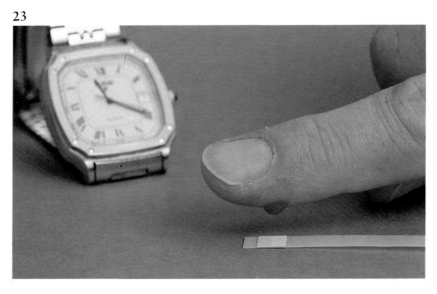

23   The period of contact between the blood and the reagent pad must be accurately timed.

24 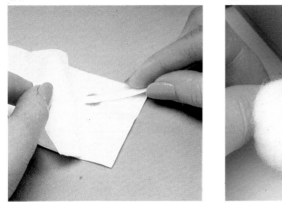 **25**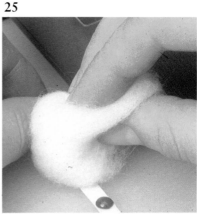

24 and 25   The blood can be wiped or blotted off the stick at the end of the carefully timed reaction.

26

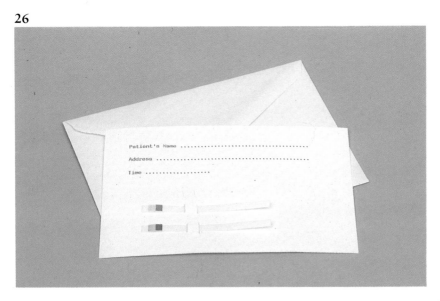

26   Used BG strips can easily be posted to the nearest hospital or laboratory for checking by the physician that the patient's diabetic control is acceptable, and that the test is being correctly carried out.

6   The enzyme reaction is specific for glucose. Any problems in the use of BG strips usually result from failure to adhere to the instructions.

7   The performance of the strip and the technique of the user can be checked with a suitable quality-control system organised through a local diabetic clinic or hospital laboratory (see **36**).

8   BG strips are designed for use with fresh capillary blood. Blood collected in a test-tube containing preservative may have a sufficiently high proportion of fluoride in solution to inhibit the reaction, and therefore BG strips should not be used to test stored blood.

9   BG strips are not advised for the assessment of the degree of hypoglycaemia, or for the assessment of the ill diabetic, as the strips are affected by ketoacidosis, which may be present with unremarkable blood glucose levels.

Interpretation of BG strips

BG STRIPS

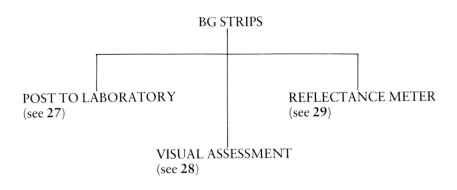

POST TO LABORATORY
(see **27**)

REFLECTANCE METER
(see **29**)

VISUAL ASSESSMENT
(see **28**)

27

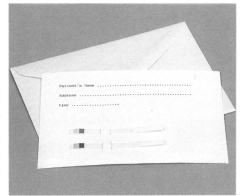

27 Assessment by post. The used strips can be sent by post, suitably labelled, to the nearest diabetic clinic or laboratory, where they can be visually assessed or read in a reflectance meter. In addition to allowing the physician to keep an eye on the patient's blood sugar levels, it is also possible to assess the adequacy of the blood collection by examining the used strips.

Precision: ± 2 mmol/l.

Range: 1 mmol/l (20 mg%) to 22 mmol/l (400 mg%) with some limited assessment up to 44 mmol/l (800 mg%).

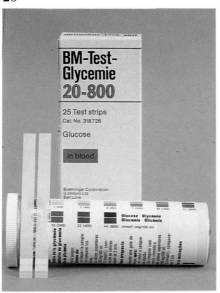

28 Visual assessment. The BG strips intended for visual assessment have double test areas, which give a colour range wider than the single test area strips. The latter are generally now used only in reflectance meters. It is extremely important that the patient is trained in the accurate reading of these colour mats and understands fully the two-colour system (see 'Quality control' and 'Colour vision'). Visual assessment by the patient can also be coupled with posting the strips to the laboratory as an additional check on the validity of the result.

29 Assessment by reflectance meter. Many small battery-powered reflectance meters are available to read BG strips. These meters are now stable and produce a fairly precise result when used in conjunction with a very carefully performed BG strip technique. As the machines are usually calibrated at the factory they rely considerably on the stability of manufacture of the BG strips for their performance.
Precision: ± 0.5 mmol/l.
Range: 3 mmol/l (60 mg%) to 22 mmol/l (400 mg%). Colour development above 22 mmol/l (400 mg%) is non-linear and therefore cannot be assessed by a simple linear calibration reflectance meter. A badly timed or badly applied BG strip will give a false sense of precision when it obtains a numerical result on one of these meters. The cost of the meters is such that they are of practical use only to high-risk diabetics.

29a

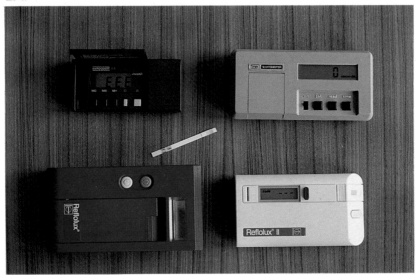

29b

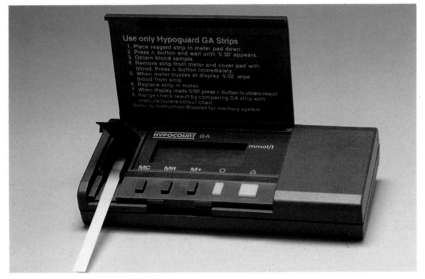

Special features obtainable in reflectance meters (30 to 32)

30

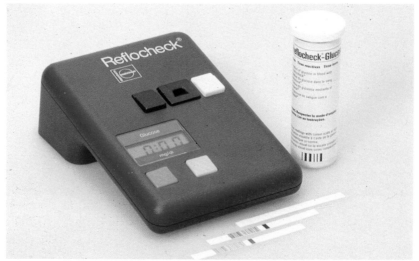

30 An expensive, high-precision, 'clinic' reflectance meter using special BG strips with a bar code to auto-zero the machine.
Precision: ± 0.2 mmol/l when used by a trained technician.

31 Meter using a twin-colour pad BG strip.
Range: 3 to 22 mmol/l. Zero is set by the bar code.

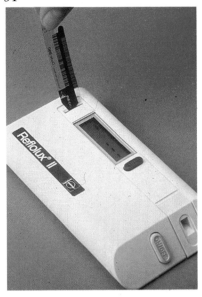

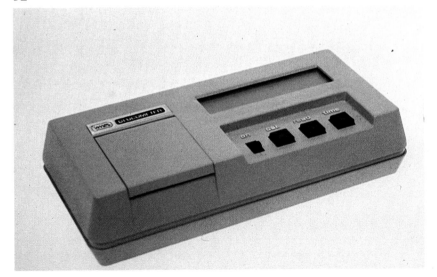

32 This meter has a memory that can recall the last 26 results.

Home blood glucose measurement for the blind diabetic

Small finger guides to enable the blind diabetic to apply a drop of blood on to a BG strip are available or can be made at low cost (33). The strip can then be inserted into a reflectance meter which produces an audible result (34). This allows blind diabetics a degree of independence in controlling their therapy. However, like all such systems, fastidious attention to technique is necessary for valid results.

33

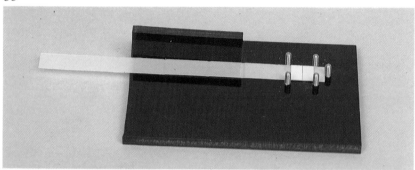

33 Finger guide to help blind diabetics place their drop of blood accurately on the BG strip.

34

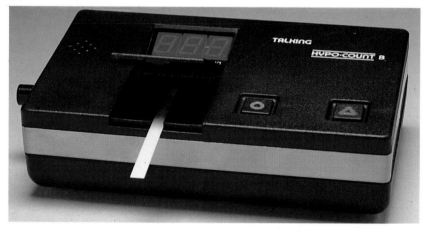

34 BG strip reflectance meter with voice synthesiser for use by the blind.

Quality control

Colour vision in the diabetic
Correct assessment of the BG strip depends upon the patient's discrimination of colour changes on the small reactant pads. Disturbances of colour vision are known in diabetics and it is therefore wise to check patients' colour acuity before allowing them to start monitoring their blood glucose at home (**35**).

35

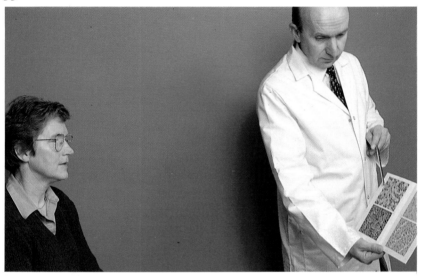

35   Testing a patient's colour vision is essential to ensure that he or she can interpret colour charts and strip tests.

Quality control schemes
All analytical systems in the laboratory or at home should be checked periodically using substances of known glucose concentration. Such quality control checks, which are part of the normal laboratory routine, should also be extended to the patient's home by providing suitable solutions that the patients treat as they would their own blood samples. They should then send the assessment of the result (or the stick that was used) to the clinic for checking.

The blood sugar result obtained by the strip method is lower than that obtained with serum and therefore the use of simple glucose solutions is valid only if they are first calibrated using the same stick technique in the laboratory. It is usually easiest to use one of the commercially manufactured solutions specifically made for use with BG strips (36).

36

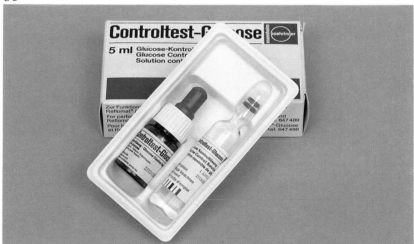

36 Example of quality control materials suitable for use in monitoring BG strip and meter performance.

4. Glycosylated haemoglobin and other proteins

The measurement of glycosylated haemoglobin is widely accepted as an objective and quantitative index of blood glucose levels during the preceding six to ten weeks, and is therefore increasingly being used in the management of patients with diabetes. Other proteins are also glycosylated non-enzymatically, and it has been shown that both glycosylated albumin and glycosylated plasma protein levels respond more quickly than those of glycosylated haemoglobin to changes in overall glycaemia, so that they too are being used in assessing control of hyperglycaemia.

The value of having these measurements made at intervals in diabetics is enormous, in that it allows special attention to be concentrated on those patients with poor control, and it also gives encouragement to both patient and doctor when normoglycaemia is being achieved and maintained.

Glycosylated haemoglobin

If haemoglobin is subjected to separation by cation exchange chromatography, a heterogeneous fast fraction separates ahead of haemoglobin A_0. Under suitable conditions, this fast fraction can be separated into haemoglobin $A1a_1$, haemoglobin $A1a_2$, haemoglobin $A1b$ and haemoglobin $A1c$. These haemoglobins elute ahead of haemoglobin A_0 and in the normal adult comprise approximately 0.2, 0.2, 0.4 and 4 to 6% of total haemoglobin respectively. (See Table 2 overleaf.)

Table 2 Composition of haemoglobins in normal adults.

Haemoglobin subunit	Subunit structure	Modification	Content
HbA_0	$\alpha_2\beta_2$		>90%
HbA_2	$\alpha_2\delta_2$		<1.5%
HbF	$\alpha_2\gamma_2$		<0.8%
HbA_1 a$_1$	$\alpha_2(\beta\text{–F–D–P})_2$	Fructose-1, 6-diphosphate	ca. 0.4%
a$_2$	$\alpha_2 (\beta\text{–G–6–P})_2$	Glucose-6, phosphate	
b	?	?Deamidation product of HbA_0	0.4%
c	$\alpha_2(\beta\text{–G})_2$	Glucose	4 to 6%
d	?	? Hb + oxidised glutathione	Trace
e	?	?	

These components (except HbA_2 and F) arise from non-enzymatic post-translational modifications of the parent haemoglobin. Haemoglobin A1c results when the terminal group of valine of the beta chain forms an aldimine adduct with glucose (in its straight chain form, which is 0.3% of total glucose).

Aldimine (pre-A_{1c})   Ketoamine (stable HbA_{1c})

This aldimine adduct can rearrange to form a more stable ketoamine. The reaction also occurs on alpha chain amino termini as well as on

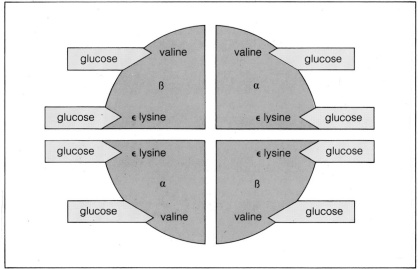

37 Diagrammatic scheme of sites of glycosylation in a haemoglobin molecule.

E amino groups of lysine on both chains, but it is only on the beta valine amino group that there is sufficient pK change to create a distinct chromatographic entity at pH values near 7 (37).

Methods of analysis of glycosylated haemoglobin that detect the glucose/haemoglobin bond will, however, also detect these non-beta valine amino forms of glycosylated haemoglobin. Haemoglobin A1c is the only fast chromatographic fraction changed by diabetes.

Methods of analysis of glycosylated haemoglobin

Ion exchange chromatography by disposable column (38)

Developments in ion exchange chromatography continue to simplify the technique of detection of haemoglobin A1c as a separate fraction. All the available techniques are specific for the beta valine group substitution amongst the glycosylated ketoamine bonds. The degree of control needed over the elution from the ion exchange column of a haemoglobin sample load depends on whether one wishes to obtain a total 'fast fraction' (haemoglobin A1a, A1b and A1c), or whether the specific quantification of haemoglobin A1c is required. Small columns of ion exchange resin are commercially available and provide quantification of the total fast fraction of haemoglobin at a modest unit cost and with very low hardware costs. (Specific quantitation of HbA1c requires a system to control elution that is usually achieved only in high performance liquid chromatography systems.)

Elution of the 'fast fraction' followed by HbA_0 is achieved with buffers of very precisely controlled pH and ionic strength. The optical density of the eluents is read in a spectrophotometer at 415 nm, and the results

38

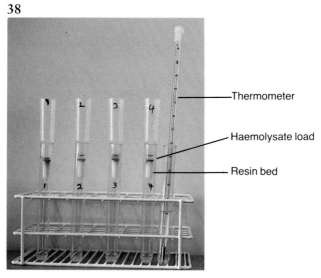

38 Four different blood samples being eluted on small disposable ion exchange columns.

expressed as a percentage ratio. The method is very temperature-dependent and either a temperature correction must be made to the values, or the elution carried out in a temperature-controlled environment.

Precision:
CV approximately 6%.

Interferences:
Interference from haemoglobin F and haemoglobinopathies can occur.

Electrophoresis and electroendosmosis (39 and 40)
These systems separate the fast fractions of haemoglobin from the main haemoglobin A_0 as a single band on agar gel plates. The plate is prepared by pouring gel on to a transparent flexible backing and the plates are run in special cells attached to a standard laboratory electrophoresis power pack. Following electrophoresis (taking approximately 45 minutes) the plates can be dried and without further treatment the two haemoglobin fractions are quantified in a suitable densitometer by scanning at 420 nm. It is necessary that the gel and the electrophoresis buffers are prepared to a very high standard of quality control. This can be done in the user's

39

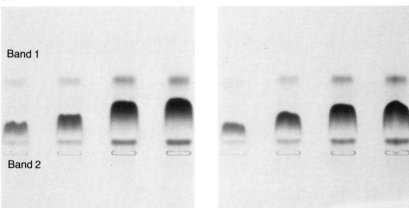

39 Two haemoglobin samples, each run in a series of dilutions, showing the load effect distorting the ratio between band 1 (the fast fraction) and band 2 (the main haemoglobin fraction). Plate stained with Coomassie blue.

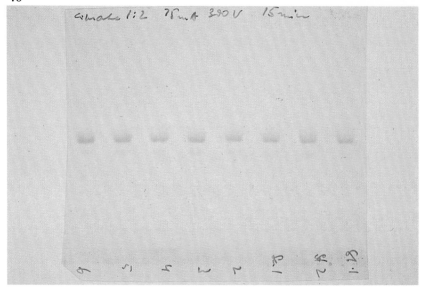

40 Unstained agar plates with samples from seven patients and one quality control sample. Note the difficulty in checking the run because of the very pale haemoglobin colour. Compare with **39**.

laboratory, but it is more often achieved by purchasing the gels and buffers as a commercial kit.

The system is slightly temperature-dependent but very load-dependent, i.e. the percentage of fast fraction is partially related to the total amount of haemoglobin loaded at the origin of the gel. The preparation of the haemolysate therefore has to be carefully done and, in addition, if the patient's haemoglobin level varies much from normal the result will be distorted.

Precision:
CV approximately 6%.

Interferences:
Haemoglobin F and some abnormal haemoglobins run as a fast fraction on this system, and are not distinguishable from haemoglobin A_{1c}. As the method does not separate haemoglobin A_{1c} from other fast fractions it cannot in itself detect haemoglobin F or any other haemoglobinopathy.

The method should therefore not be used in situations where abnormal haemoglobins are suspected.

Chemical detection of glycosylated haemoglobin

In 1976 Flückiger and Winterhalter published a method for chemical detection of glycosylated haemoglobin based on the production of a yellow colour by the interaction of 5-hydroxymethylfurfural with 2-thiobarbituric acid. The 5-hydroxymethylfurfural is produced by mild acid digestion of the glycosylated haemoglobin. Gottschalk showed in 1952 that the formation of 5-hydroxymethylfurfural under mild acid digestion is a specific test for 1-amino, 1-deoxy, 2-ketoses. The adaptation of this method by Flückiger thus gives a test for the ketoamine link of glucose to haemoglobin on any of the haemoglobin tetramers either on the valine or lysine residues.

a) Manual method (Flückiger and Winterhalter 1976)
This method, which requires calibration either with hydroxymethylfurfural itself or with precalibrated haemoglobin samples, is inexpensive but difficult to run with acceptable precision on a routine basis.

Sample size:
1 ml.

Precision:
CV 10%.

Interferences:
Glucose or fructose in large amounts.

b) Automated method
Automation of the Flückiger method allows greater precision. The method still requires external calibration and careful technical attention to detail, but provides a reasonable level of performance and a large sample-handling capacity.

Sample size:
1 ml.

Precision:
CV 5%.

Interferences:
As manual method.

High performance liquid chromatography (41 to 43)
The development of hard ion exchange gels that are capable of with-standing the pressures in an HPLC system has enabled the specific separation of haemoglobin A_{1c} by high performance chromatography to be used as a routine service technique. Several dedicated systems are available, all giving a high degree of precision and specific quantification of haemoglobin A_{1c} in a very small sample of blood. Haemoglobin F can normally be easily distinguished from the haemoglobin A_{1c} peak, and most haemoglobinopathies are also easily seen on the resultant chromatograms. These systems are expensive, but their running costs are no greater than some of the less precise systems.

41

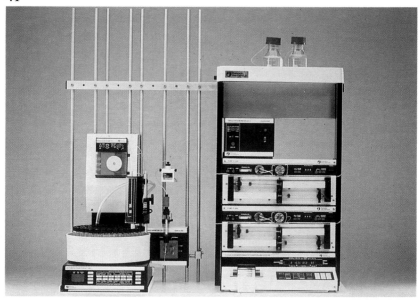

41 HPLC with autosampler and mono S column programmed to perform haemoglobin A_{1c} separations on diluted haemolysed blood samples placed on sampler turntable.

42

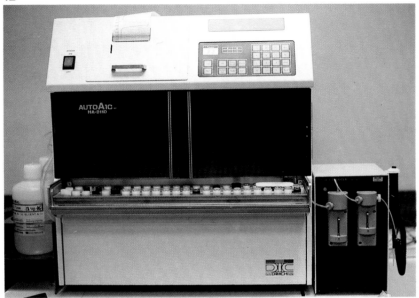

43

42 Dedicated HbA$_{1c}$ analyser capable of automatically separating and quantifying HbA$_{1c}$ by ion exchange chromatography on diluted patients' samples.

43 **Highly automated ion exchange chromatography analyser for HbA$_{1c}$ separations.** Its general performance is similar to the analysers shown in **41** and **42**.

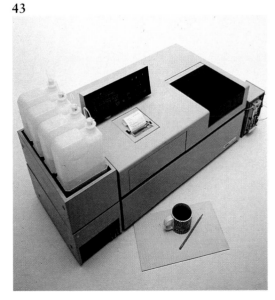

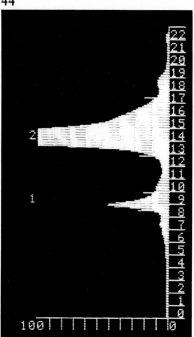

44 Example of HPLC separation of HbA$_{1c}$ (peak 1) from HbA$_0$ (peak 2).

45

```
PEAK NO.         2
PEAK MONITOR  1
RETENTION    9.99   ML
DURATION     6.89   ML
AREA         686.5  %ML
             84.66  %AA
MONITOR 1    458.0  %FS
MONITOR 2    0.0    %FS
BASELINE     7.5    %FS

PEAK NO.         1
PEAK MONITOR  1
RETENTION    5.96   ML
DURATION     2.29   ML
AREA         73.21  %ML
             9.02   %AA
MONITOR 1    75.0   %FS
MONITOR 2    0.0    %FS
BASELINE     7.5    %FS

METHOD NO.       4
RUN NO.         99
LOOP NO.         3
ACC AREA     810.9  %ML
```

45 Example of integrator printout of HPLC separation of haemoglobin A$_{1c}$ showing that the HbA$_{1c}$ (peak 1) is 9.02% of the total haemoglobin load.

46 Similar illustration to 45, showing the high degree of resolution of minor haemoglobins that can be obtained using HPLC, with haemoglobins A_{1a}, A_{1b} and haemoglobin F as well as haemoglobin A_{1c} detected in the separation.

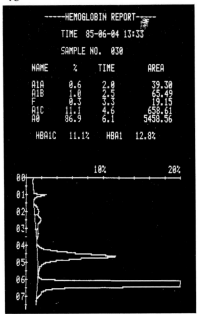

Boronic acid column chromatography

This method detects the glucose/haemoglobin link by affinity chromatography. It has much to commend it, having a specific affinity for the glucose–protein bond, but there has been some concern about variation in the resin leading to differences between sample results when the batch of resin is changed. The method is similar in cost to ion exchange chromatography.

Glycosylated serum proteins

Serum proteins are glycosylated in a similar way to haemoglobin. The half-life of serum proteins (almost half of which is albumin) is much shorter than that of haemoglobin and therefore measurement of the percentage of glycosylation of such proteins will provide information about diabetic control over a shorter period of time than is possible with glycosylated haemoglobin. Many of the methods for measuring glycosylated plasma protein are derived from glycosylated haemoglobin methodology, but an additional step of colorimetric complexing of the separated glycosylated and non-glycosylated protein fractions is necessary. With some of these glycosylated plasma protein measurements, therefore, it is difficult to maintain a sufficiently high level of precision for the results to reflect the changes in plasma glucose with any degree of sensitivity. However, two more recent methods have been developed which claim useful precision:

Automated thiobarbituric acid glycated protein determination

Precision:
CV 10%.

Comment:
Useful if the glycosylated Hb method is also being run on the same equipment.

Reference:
Moore et al. 1986.

Fructosamine assay
A dye reduction assay using nitroblue tetrazolium – simple to perform.

Precision:
CV 5%.

Comment:
Assay has considerable potential.

Reference:
Johnson et al. 1982.

5. Serum electrolytes, blood gases, osmolality and anion gap

In metabolic crises where dehydration and loss of sodium and potassium occur, ketoacidosis can develop rapidly, and where a moderately hyperosmolar state is present, measurements of serum electrolytes, arterial blood pH and blood osmolality are all important. Detection of ketosis from the breath, if one is able to smell ketones effectively (people vary in this ability), is useful as there is no delay in getting the result! The presence of urinary ketones in an ill diabetic is suggestive of ketoacidosis, though very ill patients may pass no urine when first seen. In that case a serum ketone estimation, however crude, is of value in making the diagnosis of ketoacidosis.

Estimation of serum bicarbonate levels may help when blood gas measurement is not available; arterial blood pH measurement is more useful in the ill patient.

Serum sodium and potassium levels can be normal initially in dehydrated patients despite severe depletion, but will fall rapidly with rehydration unless enough sodium chloride and potassium chloride are given. Rehydration is normally achieved with isotonic saline so that sodium replacement is usually adequate. Serum potassium levels, however, must be monitored carefully during the treatment of ketoacidosis so that potassium replacement can be given once levels fall to normal during rehydration, and can be cut back if urine output is low or if a sudden rise in blood level occurs once intracellular potassium replacement has been achieved.

Ketoacids and lactic acid can be measured specifically, and this is useful in the diagnosis of acidotic illness in diabetics if it can be done quickly. When such tests are not available, however, the severity of acid overload can be assessed objectively by the size of the anion gap, i.e. serum $(Na^+ + K^+) - (HCO_3^- + Cl^-)$. Normally the difference is less than 20, but it can rise to greater than 40 mmol/l in acidosis.

It is helpful to ascertain the plasma osmolality, as a severe hyperosmolar state can develop with ketoacidosis and severe hyperglycaemia, and this can lead to secondary diffuse intravascular coagulation. There is also a risk that during treatment of severe hyperosmolality, cerebral oedema may develop as a result of incautious rehydration. It is therefore helpful to know if plasma osmolality is nearing 320 mmols or more. If no osmometer is available it can be calculated as 2 (Na^+ + K^+) + urea + glucose in mmol/l.

In long-term management, measurement of ketoacids and lactic acids has proved useful in assessing the adequacy of various insulin replacement regimes, but these are rarely used for day-to-day patient care. Parenchymal diabetic renal disease leads to progessive renal failure and the rate of progression in the individual can be determined by plotting the inverse of the serum creatinine with time. This slope can then be used to predict when renal replacement therapy may need to be considered in an individual patient. Blood urea levels can be helpful but are less objective because of upsets resulting from current diet, hydration and acute illness.

Laboratory tests for disturbances of blood gas and electrolyte metabolism

Blood gas determinations

In a metabolic diabetic crisis it is necessary to have a facility for the precise measurement of blood gases and pH. Other tests of acid base disturbance described later are usually of second choice and are used only in the absence of such equipment.

Blood gas analysers measure directly pH, P_{CO_2} and P_{O_2}. They also usually calculate values derived from these three measurements such as:

Actual bicarbonate, which is calculated from the Henderson Hasselbach equation, e.g. $pH = 6.1 + log \dfrac{[HCO_3^-]}{P_{CO_2} + 0.23}$

Standard bicarbonate is calculated from the same equation but uses a P_{CO_2} value in the middle of the normal range. This 'standardised' value is an estimate of the bicarbonate in the patient, assuming any respiratory abnormality to have been corrected. This practical concept separates disturbances of acid base metabolism into respiratory and non-respiratory. (For further details readers should consult a textbook on acid base metabolism.)

In a metabolic crisis in a diabetic the following defects are seen:

1   Low pH – metabolic acidosis caused by gross excess of ketone bodies and sometimes by lactate.

2   Low P_{CO_2} – respiratory compensation for the metabolic acidosis. As this is a compensatory effect it may not be seen in patients who have

56

become extremely ill very quickly, or in patients with a compromised respiratory system.

3 PO_2 largely unchanged unless there is concomitant respiratory pathology.

Arterial blood must be used for determining blood gases as there is a significant difference between arterial and venous pH and PCO_2. Much of this difference results from changes that occur during tissue perfusion, and will be severely affected by any degree of peripheral collapse in a metabolic crisis. Arterial blood must be sufficiently anticoagulated with heparin to remain fluid whilst the measurement is being carried out, but an excess of heparin (which is an acid mucopolysaccharide) may lower the pH of the sample.

The blood sample, if it is to reflect accurately the metabolic state of the patient, must not be kept for long before measurement takes place, as the cells in the sample will continue to metabolise. For example, a blood sample must be kept no longer than 30 minutes at 2°C.

Blood gas analysers (47 and 48)
Many modern blood gas analysers have been developed for use in neonatal intensive care units and therefore use very small sample volumes

47

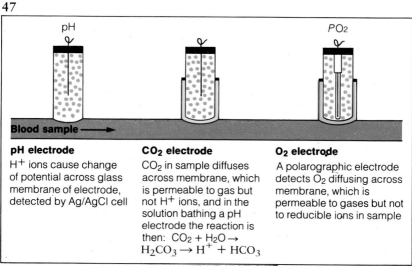

pH electrode
H⁺ ions cause change of potential across glass membrane of electrode, detected by Ag/AgCl cell

CO₂ electrode
CO₂ in sample diffuses across membrane, which is permeable to gas but not H⁺ ions, and in the solution bathing a pH electrode the reaction is then: $CO_2 + H_2O \rightarrow H_2CO_3 \rightarrow H^+ + HCO_3$

O₂ electrode
A polarographic electrode detects O₂ diffusing across membrane, which is permeable to gases but not to reducible ions in sample

47   Diagram of blood gas analyser electrodes.

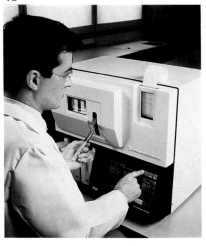

```
             174
TIME     15:09
DATE  JAN 29 1987

OPID

PTID
FIO2
TEMP    37.0       0
TYPE

HB         0.0      G%
PH         7.158
PCO2       7.15     KPA
FO2        7.46     KPA

HCO3      18.3      MM/L
ABE       -8.1      MM/L
SBC       17.5      MM/L
```

48 A syringe sample of arterial blood being loaded on to an automated blood gas analyser, and an example of the results printout.

(80 μl or less). These machines have small blood pathways which can block easily unless great care is exercised with the quality of the sample. Unless this small sample volume facility is an important clinical need, a blood gas analyser is easier to maintain if it is designed to take syringe sample volumes (200 μl).

Secondary measurement of acid base disturbance

If blood gas analysis is not available close to the patient then the following parameters can be of use:

Plasma bicarbonate

As noted earlier, the abnormality in a diabetic crisis with acidosis is caused by the production of ketone bodies or lactate. This excess hydrogen ion load is dealt with by the body in the following way:

$$HCO_3^- + H^+ \rightarrow H_2CO_3 \rightarrow CO_2 + H_2O$$

The fall in bicarbonate is therefore directly proportional to the amount of hydrogen ion neutralised.

Bicarbonate measurements by automated technology. Many multi-channel laboratory analysers include an assessment of serum bicarbonate with their electrolyte determinations. These systems often use a CO_2 electrode (as described for the blood gas analyser) but before the sample is presented to the electrode it is treated with weak acid to liberate the CO_2 from the bicarbonate. The electrode then measures the total CO_2 in the sample i.e. CO_2 and HCO_3. Such an automated bicarbonate measurement should be precise to $\pm$ 2 mmol/l and should be a good secondary method of assessing the patient's metabolic balance. It also has the advantage that the measurement can be carried out on venous blood.

Alternative methods of bicarbonate determination. Sometimes the physical distance of the main laboratory from the acutely ill patient or the inability of such a laboratory to provide a true 24-hour service makes alternative methods of assessing bicarbonate necessary. Of these methods the simplest, but not necessarily the most precise, are often also based on the release of CO_2 from bicarbonate in the sample, as already described, but, by changing the proportions of acid to sample, the CO_2 is evolved as gas. The volume of CO_2 evolved can then be measured.

The Natelson microgasometer (**49**) is a gas burette, connected via a mercury-filled syringe to a reaction chamber. The sample, followed by the weak acid reagent, is presented to the sample nozzle. Measured amounts of both are drawn into the reaction chamber by manipulation of the metal plunger in the mercury syringe. The CO_2 is liberated from the sample by shaking the reaction chamber with the acid reagent. The mercury in the manometer arm is displaced and therefore gives a measurement of the volume of gas evolved. This represents the total CO_2 in the sample.

Other microgasometers are shown in **50** to **52**. These ingenious devices are simplified forms of the Natelson equipment described above. A measured volume of serum is added to the lactic acid in the reaction bottles. The bottle or cuvette is then quickly capped with the gas-tight syringe. The whole assembly is shaken and the evolved CO_2 displaces the piston in the syringe or the bubble in the capillary thereby giving an estimate of the total CO_2 evolved from the serum sample. The method is not terribly precise, but is inexpensive.

Precision:
CV approximately 10 to 15%.

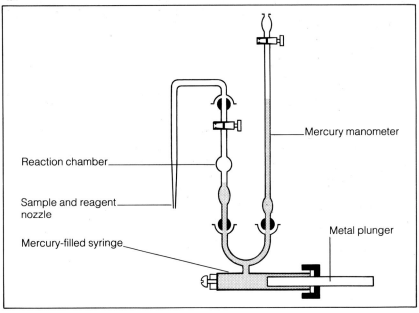

Mercury manometer

Reaction chamber

Sample and reagent
nozzle

Mercury-filled syringe

Metal plunger

49 Natelson microgasometer.

50

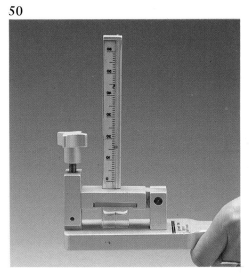

50 Example of CO_2 apparatus in use. The bicarbonate value is read off the scale by determining the height of the column of liquid in the capillary tube.

51

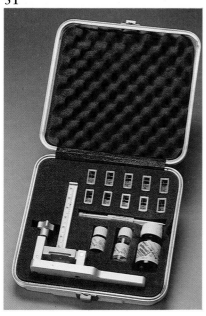

51 Same CO_2 apparatus as shown in 50, in carrying case with cuvettes for 10 bicarbonate determinations.

52

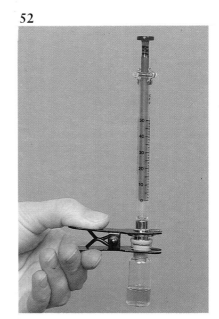

52 Alternative CO_2 apparatus.

Measurement of ketone bodies

The measurement of serum ketones (acetone, acetoacetate or ß–hydroxybutyrate) has never been developed to the same extent as that of pH and bicarbonate. Serum ketones can be estimated approximately by placing one drop of centrifuged serum or plasma on a reagent tablet. The colour change can be difficult to interpret as the serum has a yellowish colour, but if after 30 seconds a violet colour is seen the test is positive for excess ketones (53). The test should then be repeated with plasma diluted two, four and then eight times. In a normal subject there should be no colour change with undiluted plasma at 30 seconds, whilst at the other extreme, the plasma of a patient with severe diabetic ketoacidosis is usually positive at an eight-fold dilution.

53

Negative reaction

Ketoacidosis – after 30 seconds
at a quarter dilution

53 Use of reagent tablets for the detection of ketone bodies: on the left is a negative reaction, and on the right, the violet colour indicates a positive reading after 30 seconds, at ¼ dilution.

Lactic acid

Lactic acidosis can occur on its own or can complicate diabetic keto-acidosis, particularly if tissue perfusion is poor, and, in both lactic acidosis and ketoacidosis, volume depletion and hypotension can reduce glomerular filtration so that the acidosis is further aggravated by renal failure. Lactate can be measured enzymatically in a general laboratory. However, this measurement should be secondary to assessing the response to treatment of the patient's metabolic crisis by pH or bicarbonate measurements.

Sodium and potassium determinations

Physiological control mechanisms in the body strive to keep the ionic activity of sodium and potassium in the body water at a constant level. In hyperproteinaemia or hyperlipidaemia the concentration of ions in the total volume of the blood sample will be reduced but the concentration of ions in the water is normal. Hyperlipidaemia in diabetic ketoacidosis can thus interfere with the measurement of sodium and potassium in this manner and produce falsely low values. This error does not usually create a clinical problem with potassium because the normal range is large with respect to the concentration in serum, for example a reference range of 3.5 to 5 mmol/l represents a change of over 33% in concentration. Sodium, however, has a reference range of 135 to 145 mmol/l, representing only a 7% change in concentration.

This interference is seen in plasma emission spectrophotometry as the result relates to the total volume of the sample; it is also seen with ion-selective electrodes based on indirect methods, where the sample is initially diluted, the dilution depending on the volume measurements of the total original sample. Direct ion-selective electrodes, i.e. using non-diluted samples, measure ionic activity in the sample water and are therefore not subject to interference in this way. The interference from lipid can be removed by prolonged centrifugation before measurement by flame photometry or indirect ion-selective electrode measurement. Interference from hyperproteinaemia can be dealt with only by direct ion-selective electrode measurement. Equipment for the measurement of sodium and potassium by both emission spectrophotometry and indirect and direct ion-selective electrodes is currently available from many manufacturers (54 to 57).

54

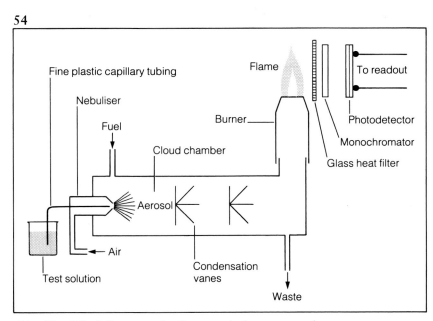

54   Simplified diagram of a flame-emission spectrophotometer.

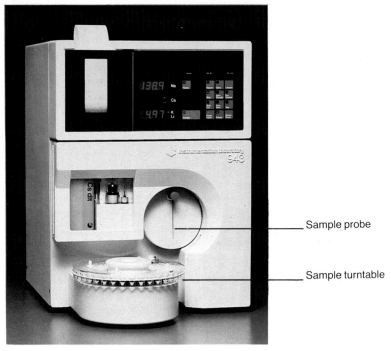

Sample probe

Sample turntable

55 Automated flame-emission spectrophotometer with multi-sample turntable.

Ion-selective electrodes (56 and 57)
This method uses a glass ion-exchange membrane for sodium, and a valinomycin neutral carrier membrane for potassium measurement. Typical sodium electrodes have 1,000-fold greater selectivity for sodium than potassium, and typical potassium electrodes have a 10,000-fold greater selectivity for potassium than sodium. Both electrodes are insensitive to pH.

Precision:
CV 5%.

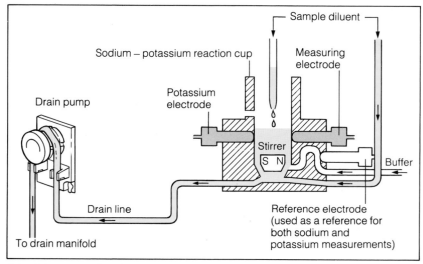

56 Diagram of indirect ion-selective electrodes for measuring sodium and potassium.

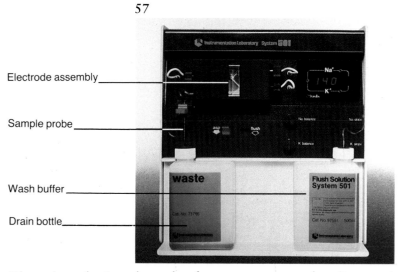

57 Direct ion-selective electrodes for measurement of sodium and potassium.

Osmolality

Osmolality is the term used to identify the number of moles of solute particles per kilogram of water. This definition depends not on the kind of particles but only on their number.

This measurement can either be calculated using a formula dependent on direct measurement of the most osmotically active particles in the sample, or by direct measurement, because of the physical properties of the osmotically active particles.

Direct measurement or osmometry
There are two methods. In the first, the propensity of solute to lower the freezing point of water is used. In the osmometer the degree of depression of the freezing point in the sample compared with pure water is an estimate of the amount of solute in the serum sample. The equipment is calibrated with salt solutions of known sodium chloride content (58).

Precision:
CV 10%.

A second form of osmometer (capable of accepting very small samples) depends on vapour pressure depression. However, if ketoacids are present in gross excess in the serum of diabetics, these contribute to the

58

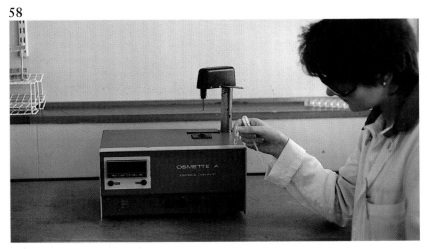

58   Freezing point osmometer.

vapour pressure of the water and interfere with the results. Vapour pressure osmometry should not therefore be used in diabetic ketoacidosis.

Calculation of osmolality and anion gap

Calculation of the plasma osmolality by the sum of the major ions present in the plasma can be a useful alternative to direct measurement. The simple calculation is described on page 56, and is sometimes part of the programme package in a multichannel laboratory analyser, which uses the analytical results from the sample to produce the calculated osmolality. In addition, the severity of acid overload in a patient can be roughly calculated by the sum of the major anions minus that of the major cations, which can either be calculated by the clinician or can be included as part of the electrolyte analyser programme. These calculations can be of great use clinically in the absence of direct specific measurements, provided the clinician remembers that the results are approximations and cannot have the precision of direct laboratory measurements.

6. Hyperlipidaemia in diabetes mellitus

Hyperlipidaemia is a feature of life in the western world and carries with it increased risks of vascular diseases. Diabetes mellitus increases or accelerates these risks, and the degree of risk probably increases with worsening control of glycaemia. Secondary hypertriglyceridaemia is seen with poor control and can be corrected by a few days of normo-glycaemia. Hypercholesterolaemia has a less clear-cut relationship to glycaemia in diabetics. This may be because levels are slower to change and because relationships of the various individual lipid transport materials to glycaemia are not well defined. In general, high-density lipoprotein (HDL) cholesterol, believed to protect against atheroma, tends to be low, and low-density lipoprotein (LDL) cholesterol tends to be raised with prolonged hyperglycaemia in diabetes. Some reasons for this are known. For example, glycosylated LDL cholesterol, which is increased by hyperglycaemia, cannot be recognised by its cellular receptors, so cholesterol fails to get into cells where normally its internalization would both 'switch off' cholesterol synthesis and lead to degradation of the cholesterol entering the cell.

Value of lipid measurements
Measurement of triglycerides is useful in assessing short-term changes in glycaemia. Measurement of cholesterol-bearing proteins is best done only after glycaemia has been corrected (as far as possible) for several weeks, so that hyperlipidaemia requiring additional specific treatment can be identified and not confused with the secondary hyperlipidaemia induced by the diabetes itself.

Lipids in diabetes mellitus

Plasma lipids are a heterogeneous group of compounds classified by their hydrophobic nature and large molecular size. They repel water and so resist being solubilised in water or aqueous solutions. The transport of lipids to and from body tissues is accomplished by complexing the hydrophobic lipid with a hydrophillic compound such as a phospholipid or an aproprotein. The resultant lipoprotein is then capable of transporting the lipid throughout the circulatory system.

There are four types of lipoprotein: each type has a different proportion of triglyceride and cholesterol (59).

Triglycerides

Triglycerides are complexes of glycerol and fatty acids. They are present in chylomicrons and very low-density lipoproteins (VLDL). The usual method of analysis involves splitting the glycerol from the fatty acid moiety and then measuring the glycerol enzymatically.

The separation of dietary triglycerides contained in chylomicra from endogenous liver triglycerides contained in the very low-density lipoprotein is achieved by fasting the patient to clear the serum of the dietary component.

Triglyceride (triolein)

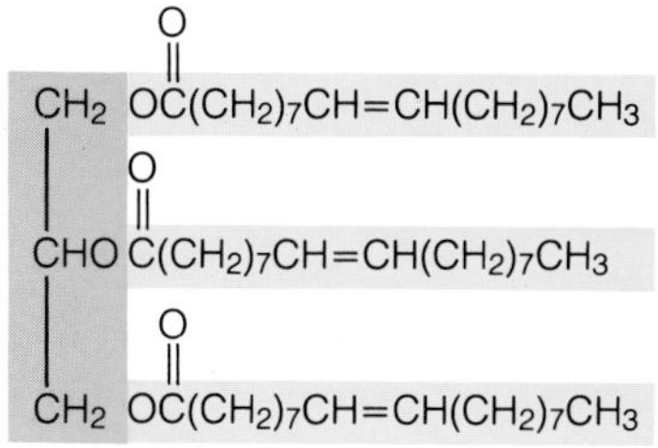

$$CH_2 \quad OC(CH_2)_7CH=CH(CH_2)_7CH_3$$
$$CHO \quad C(CH_2)_7CH=CH(CH_2)_7CH_3$$
$$CH_2 \quad OC(CH_2)_7CH=CH(CH_2)_7CH_3$$

▨ Glycerol residue   ▢ Fatty acid

Cholesterol

Cholesterol is a ring structure chemically described as a perhydrocyclopentantholine. It circulates both as free cholesterol and cholesterol ester, and is present in the lipoprotein groups LDL (low-density lipoprotein) and HDL (high-density lipoprotein).(See 59.)

Cholesterol

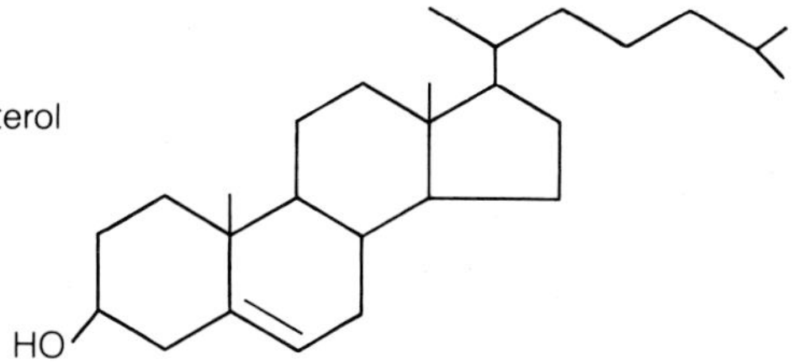

HO

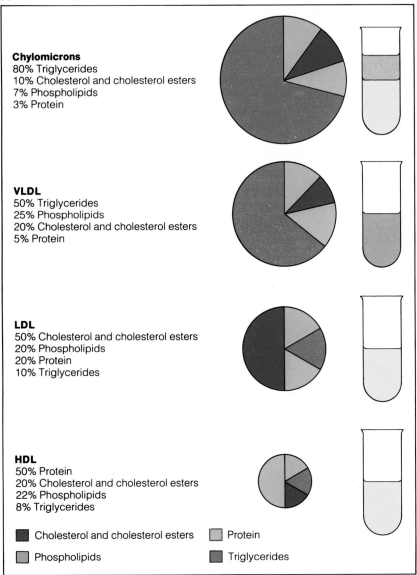

Chylomicrons
80% Triglycerides
10% Cholesterol and cholesterol esters
7% Phospholipids
3% Protein

VLDL
50% Triglycerides
25% Phospholipids
20% Cholesterol and cholesterol esters
5% Protein

LDL
50% Cholesterol and cholesterol esters
20% Phospholipids
20% Protein
10% Triglycerides

HDL
50% Protein
20% Cholesterol and cholesterol esters
22% Phospholipids
8% Triglycerides

Cholesterol and cholesterol esters   Protein

Phospholipids   Triglycerides

59 Diagrammatic representation of the percentage of constituents in lipoprotein classes and their appearance in serum when present in excess.

Analysis

Cholesterol and triglyceride can be measured using dry reagent (stick) technology or conventional laboratory wet chemistry systems. Unlike triglyceride, very little of the circulating cholesterol-containing lipoprotein is immediately derived from the diet and therefore fasting will not aid the separation of these fractions.

The separation of the two main cholesterol-containing lipoproteins can be accomplished only in the laboratory, usually by using selective precipitation techniques. These techniques enable the low-density lipoprotein and high-density lipoprotein to be analysed separately for their cholesterol content. Interest in the separation of these two fractions has stemmed from the belief that high-density lipoprotein is a protective factor in the development of atheromatous change, as it is concerned in transporting cholesterol away from peripheral tissues to the liver for excretion.

Quality control

Quality control of lipid determinations is very important. Dry chemistry systems, being used mostly in clinics and on the ward, must be incorporated in an organised quality control system if the results are to justify clinical confidence. In addition, lipid control in a patient requires long-term method stability against which to measure any change.

Quality control materials of animal origin can have relatively low native cholesterol and triglyceride values, but many modern animal sera are altered to produce a useful high range of values and can therefore be used for quality control of lipid methods.

Triglyceride analysis

Analysis should be carried out on a specimen obtained following a 14-hour fast so that no triglyceride derived from the diet is present in circulating chylomicra. As with cholesterol, chemical triglyceride analysis is obsolete. Wet and dry chemistry systems are enzyme based.

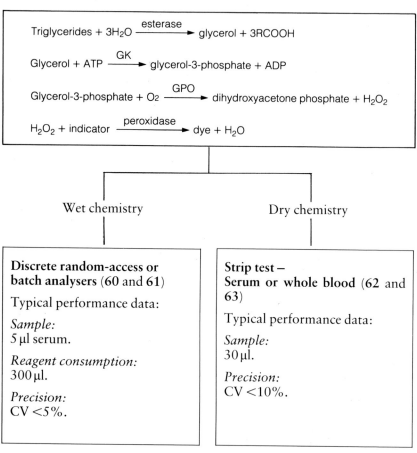

Triglycerides + $3H_2O$ $\xrightarrow{\text{esterase}}$ glycerol + 3RCOOH

Glycerol + ATP $\xrightarrow{\text{GK}}$ glycerol-3-phosphate + ADP

Glycerol-3-phosphate + O_2 $\xrightarrow{\text{GPO}}$ dihydroxyacetone phosphate + H_2O_2

H_2O_2 + indicator $\xrightarrow{\text{peroxidase}}$ dye + H_2O

Wet chemistry

Dry chemistry

Discrete random-access or batch analysers (60 and 61)

Typical performance data:

Sample:
5 μl serum.

Reagent consumption:
300 μl.

Precision:
CV <5%.

**Strip test –
Serum or whole blood (62 and 63)**

Typical performance data:

Sample:
30 μl.

Precision:
CV <10%.

Total cholesterol analysis

Chemical methods of cholesterol analysis are now obsolete. They involve the use of strong mineral acids and produce uneven colour reaction rates for free and esterified cholesterol fractions in serum. There is also marked interference by nonspecific chromogens and by bilirubin.

Enzymatic cholesterol analysis

Wet and dry chemistry systems use the same enzyme sequence and differ only in their final dye complexing steps.

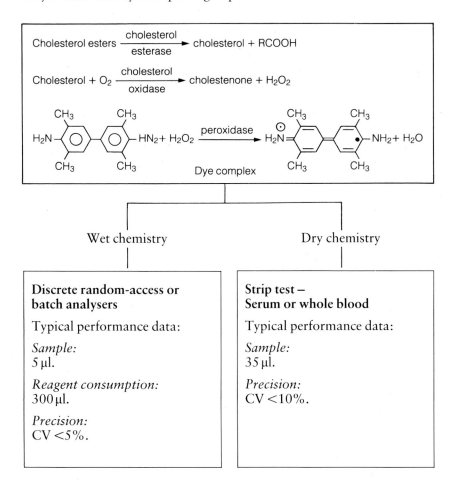

Wet chemistry

Dry chemistry

Discrete random-access or batch analysers

Typical performance data:

Sample:
5 µl.

Reagent consumption:
300 µl.

Precision:
CV <5%.

**Strip test –
Serum or whole blood**

Typical performance data:

Sample:
35 µl.

Precision:
CV <10%.

60

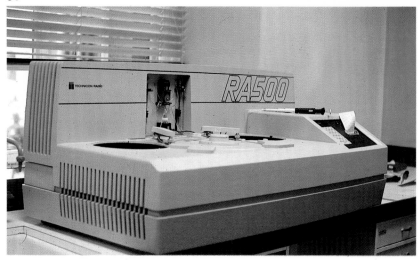

60   Discrete random access analyser designed to carry out multiple tests on the same sample.

61

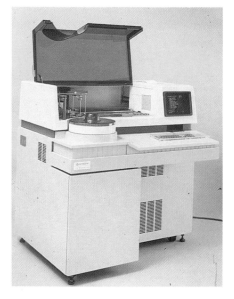

61 Analyser of large work capacity providing approximately **300 results per hour** for batches of the same test.

62

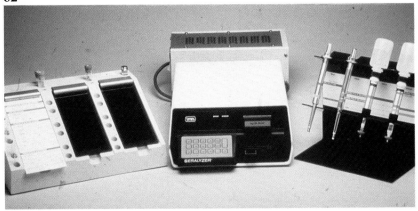

62 Dry strip-based analyser system for cholesterol detection, using serum.

63

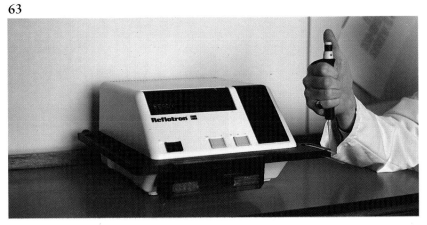

63 Dry strip-based analyser system for cholesterol detection, using whole blood.

7. Other monitoring techniques

Serum phosphate
Phosphate depletion, suspected as serum levels fall to <0.6 mmol/l, is thought to impair the release of energy from adenosine triphosphate (ATP) in cells. If phosphate replacement is shown to improve outcome in the treatment of ketoacidosis, then early measurement may become important. (See page 77.)

Fibrin degradation products
Tests should be done for diffuse intravascular coagulation if mental alertness diminishes with treatment in metabolic crises, if coma is present or persists, or if purpura appears. Total platelets will fall and fragments may be seen on blood films. Fibrin degradation products will rise, and eventually the prothrombin time increases. (See page 78.)

Tests for sepsis
The total white cell count and the percentage of polymorphonuclear leucocytes are often measured in ketoacidosis, but as a polymorphonuclear leucocytosis is usually caused by the ketoacidosis itself, this is not as helpful as careful clinical review, examination of the urine for pus and bacteria, blood cultures and chest x-ray, etc., as suggested clinically.

Serum carnitine estimation
Measurements of carnitine are unlikely to be needed routinely unless levels are shown to relate directly to problems that can be corrected. This might be the case if, for example, carnitine deficiency was shown, by reducing free fatty acid transfer to ketoacids for oxidation, to increase atheromatous disease or to relate in some other way to the increased health risks of diabetics. (See page 79.)

Polyol levels
The polyols (higher alcohols) formed from glucose in increasing amounts when it accumulates in the cells as a result of reduced glycolysis, include sorbitol, which is suspected of having a role in the production of some diabetic complications. Measurements of sorbitol levels in blood or in certain tissues may prove useful, therefore, in monitoring control or in

monitoring doses of therapeutic agents used to reduce sorbitol formation, if these come into general use. (See page 80.)

Serum phosphate measurement

The most commonly used principle is the reaction of phosphate ions with molybdate to form the complex ammoniumphosphomolybdate. This can be measured directly at 340 nm or further complexed by reducing agents to form a molybdenum blue dye. This blue compound is a complex polymer of unknown structure which is measured by spectroscopy at approximately 660 nm.

The direct measurement of unreduced ammoniumphosphomolybdate produces a faster and simpler reaction. This method has been widely adapted for modern random access and centrifugal laboratory analysers. The method should be standardised with serum as the reaction rate is different between protein-containing and simple aqueous solutions. There is no dry chemistry (stick) test for phosphate.

Interferences

Phosphate is a major intracellular anion, therefore haemolysis of the sample will cause a marked elevation of the serum result, in addition to some interference by the haemoglobin colour. Blood that has been kept for any time with the cells still in contact with the serum will also demonstrate an elevated phosphate value because of leakage of intracellular phosphate in vitro.

General reaction

$$PO_4 + H_2SO_4 + (NH_4)_6\ MO_7O_{24}\ 4H_2O \longrightarrow M_0P_{04} \quad + \text{reducing agent} \longrightarrow M^0 \text{ blue polymer complex}$$

Sample:	3 to 5 μl	5 to 10 μl
Wavelength:	340 nm with blank	varies, e.g. 620 nm no blank
Precision:	CV 5%	CV 5%

Fibrin degradation products (FDPs)

Diffuse intravascular coagulation (DIC) is a condition in which both intravascular coagulation and thrombolysis occur. The product of the thrombolysis, FDPs, when present in excess have a heparin-like effect in their own right and therefore contribute to the haemorrhagic tendency already caused by the excess thrombolysis already present as part of the condition.

Blood samples for FDP measurement must be placed in a special FDP tube, which contains reagents for accelerated clot retraction (to remove circulating fibrinogen from the sample) and a fibrinolysis inhibitor (to prevent in-vitro fibrinolysis from obscuring the result).

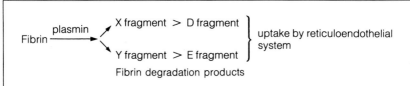

Detection by immunochemistry

a) Latex agglutination

Precision:
CV 5%.

b) Laser nephelometry

Precision:
CV 5%.

Carnitine

Carnitine catalyses the transfer of activated long-chain fatty acids across mitochondrial membrane before oxidation in the matrix of the mitochondrium. Free L-carnitine is a normal component of human serum. Laboratory methods exist to measure levels in serum by microbiological assay, radioisotopic assay and by gas chromatography. The method described here, however, uses a simple chemical reaction, is reasonably precise, and can be adapted to be carried out on standard modern laboratory analysers.

L-carnitine + acetyl CoA $\longrightarrow$ acetylcarnitine + $\longrightarrow$ Thiopentolate ion (measure
(in deproteinised sample) $\longleftarrow$ CoA + DTNB* spectrophotometrically at 405 to
415 nm)

*(DTNB = 55' dithiobis 2-nitrobenzoic acid)

The serum is deproteinised with either perchloric acid (6% solution in equal volumes with serum) and careful filtration, or by boiling and freezing.

Reference:
Rodrigues-Segade, 1986.

Precision:
CV 10%.

Polyols – laboratory background

Monosaccharides may be reduced to their corresponding alcohols; thus glucose yields sorbitol, galactose yields dulcitol, mannose yields mannitol, and fructose yields both mannitol and sorbitol. The prevention of excessive accumulation of sorbitol by the use of aldose-reductase inhibitors in diabetic nephropathy, retinopathy and neuropathy is currently being investigated (see pages 76 to 77).

Methods

No side-room method has been devised for the estimation of polyols.

Although the erythrocyte is in many ways a highly atypical cell metabolically, it is the cell most easily studied. Venous blood is collected into a heparinised tube, and the erythrocytes spun down and washed in saline. The cells are then lysed and deproteinised. The polyol levels can be determined either enzymatically or by gas chromatography. In either case the amount of polyol present is expressed in relation to the grams of haemoglobin in the original sample.

Enzymatic determination of sorbitol

This determination depends on the specific activity of sorbitol dehydrogenase and the reaction of NAD to NADH. It can be monitored either fluorimetrically for maximum sensitivity or colorimetrically for simplicity. The latter is probably the method of choice, but it remains a largely research-based laboratory investigation.

Enzymatic sorbitol measurement

$$Sorbitol + NAD \xrightarrow{\text{SDH}} fructose + NADH$$

De-proteinised
red-cell lysate

Colorimeter 340 nm
fluorimeter 366 to 434 nm

(SDH = sorbitol dehydrogenase)

Precision:
CV 15%.

Gas chromatography

Gas chromatography of polyols is a labour-intensive procedure. However it will give separation of most intracellular polyols rather than just sorbitol, as measured by the enzymatic determination. This remains a research procedure.

Precision:
CV 15 to 20%.

References

Cooper GR, McDaniel V. *Standard methods in clinical chemistry 6.* New York: Academic Press, 1970: 159.

Dubowski KM. An O-toluidine method for body-fluid glucose determination. *Clin Chem* 1962; 8: 215.

Flückiger R, Winterhalter KH. In-vitro synthesis of haemoglobin A_{1c}. *FEBS Lett 71*: 1976; 356.

Gamelon TR, James HC, Batstone GF. The determination of blood spot glucose concentration using a rapid kinetic assay. *Scand J Clin Lab Invest* 1982; **42**: 643.

Gottschalk A. Some biochemically relevant properties of N-substituted fructosamines derived from N-glucosylamino-acids and N-arylglucosamines. *Biochem J* 1952: 455.

Johnson RN, Metcalf PA, Baker JR. Fructosamine: a new approach to the estimation of serum glycosylprotein. An index of diabetic control. *Clin Chim Acta* 1982; **127**: 87.

Kadish AH, Little RL, Sternberg JC. A new and rapid method for the determination of glucose by measurement of rate of oxygen consumption. *Clin Chem* 1968; **14**: 116.

Moore J, Outlaw MC, Barnes AJ, Turner RC. Glycosylated plasma protein measurement by a semi-automated method. *Ann Clin Biochem* 1986; **23**(2): 198.

Richardson T. A modification of the Trinder Autoanalyser method for glucose. *Ann Clin Biochem* 1977; **14**: 223.

Rodrigues-Segade S, de la Pena CA, Paz M, sel Rio R. Determination of L-carnitine in serum and implementation on the ABA 100 and Centrificem 600. *Clin Chem* 1986; 31(5): 754.

Trinder P. Determination of glucose in blood using glucose oxidase with an alternative oxygen acceptor. *Ann Clin Biochem* 1969; 6: 24.

Winkers PLM, Jacob PH. A simple and automated determination of glucose in body fluids using an aqueous O-toluidine acetic agent reagent. *Clin Chim Acta* 1971; 34: 401.

Acknowledgements

The authors are pleased to acknowledge the following manufacturers, some of whom provided illustrations, and others who willingly gave their permission to use illustrations of their products.

Ames (Miles Laboratories Ltd).
Bio–Rad Laboratories Ltd.
BDH Ltd.
Fiske Associates.
Hypoguard (UK) Ltd.
Kyoto Daiichi Kagaku Co. Ltd.
Pharmacia Ltd.
Technicon Instruments Co. Ltd.

Beckman–RIIC Ltd.
Boehringer Corporation Ltd.
Corning Medical.
V.A. Howe & Company Ltd.
Instrumentation Laboratory (UK) Ltd.
Owen Mumford Ltd.
Sherwood Medical.
Travenol Laboratories Ltd.

We would also like to thank the Department of Medical Illustration, University of Aberdeen for taking some of the photographs and Mrs Mary Dow for her painstaking secretarial help in the preparation of this manuscript.

Index

Flame-emission
  spectrophotometer, 63
Fructosamine assay, 54

G
Glucose, 21
– oral tolerance test, WHO
  guidelines, 21
Glucose oxidase, 9, 23-4
Glycosuria, 7-11
– copper reduction test (tablet),
  7-9
– detection by enzyme strip, 9-11
Glycosylated haemoglobin,
  43-53
– analysis methods, 46-9
– – electroendosmosis, 47-8
– – electrophoresis, 47-8
– – ion exchange
  chromatography by
  disposable column, 46-7
– boronic acid column
  chromatography, 52
– chemical detection, 49
– high performance liquid
  chromatography, 50-3
Glycosylated low-density
  lipoprotein, 68
Glycosylated serum proteins,
  53-4
– fructosamine assay, 54
– thiobarbituric glycated protein
  determination, automated, 54

H
Haemoglobin
– composition (normal adult), 44
– glycosylation sites, 45
Haemoglobin A_{1c}, 44, 45, 46
Henderson Hasselbach equation,
  56
Heparin, 57

High-density lipoprotein
  cholesterol, 68, 69-71
Hypercholesterolaemia, 68
Hyperlipidaemia, 62, 68-75
Hyperosmolality, 55
Hyperproteinaemia, 62

J
Joslin Diabetes Foundation
  Medal, 4

K
Ketoacidosis, 55
Ketones
– detection from breath, 55
– measurement, 62
– urinary, 55
Ketone-sensitive stick tests, 14
Ketone-sensitive tablets, 13
Ketonuria, 12-13

L
Lactic acid, 62
– measurements, 55, 56, 62
Leucocyte esterase, 19
Lipids, 68
– quality control, 71
– value of measurements, 68
Lipoproteins, 68-9, 70

M
Metabolic crisis, 55-7
Microgasometers, 59-61
– Natelson, 59, 60
Microproteinuria
  (microalbuminuria) detection,
  16-18
Multiple stick tests, 16-17

N
Natelson microgasometer, 59, 60

Nelson–Somogyi reaction, 22
Nitrite, urinary, 18-19

O
Ortho-toluidine, 22-3
Osmolality, 66
– calculation, 56, 67
– direct measurement, 66-7
Osmometry, 66-7

P
Phosphate, serum, 76
– measurement, 77
– – interferences, 77
Polymorphonuclear leucocytosis, 76
Polyols, 76-7, 80-1
– enzymatic determination of sorbitol, 80
– gas chromatography, 81
Potassium, serum, 55
– determination, 62-5
– – ion-selective electrodes, 64-5
Protein, normal urine content, 16
Protein/creatinine ratio, urinary albumin expressed as, 18
Proteinuria (albuminuria), 15
– detection, 15-16

R
Reagent strip tests (BG strips), 25, 28, 30-40
– assessment by post, 33, 35
– colour vision of patient, 41
– quality control, 41-2
– reflectance meter assessment, 36-9

– – blind diabetics, 40
– – twin colour pads, 36
– visual assessment, 36
Rehydration, 55
Renal disease, diabetic, 56

S
Sepsis, tests for, 76
Sodium, serum, 55
– determination, 62-5
– – ion-selective electrodes, 64-5
Sorbitol, enzymatic determination, 80
Spectrophotometer, flame-emission, 63-64

T
Thiobarbituric acid glycated protein determination, automated, 54
Triglycerides, 69
– analysis, 71, 72
– measurement, 71

U
Urea, blood levels, 56
Urinary tract infections, 18-20
Urine
– excess leucocytes, 19
– normal protein content, 16
– reducing substances, 7-9

V
Venous blood, 5

W
White cell count, 76